Copyright 2023

All right reserved.No part of this book should be reproduced without express permission of the author.

Reproduction of all or any part of this book is punishable unders relevant law.

1

Table of Contents

A hiatal hernia is when your stomach bulges up into your chest through an opening in your diaphragm, the muscle that separates the two areas. The opening is called the hiatus, so this condition is also called a hiatus hernia.

There are two main types of hiatal hernias: sliding and paraesophageal.

Ordinarily, your esophagus (food pipe) goes through the hiatus and attaches to your stomach. In a sliding hiatal hernia, your stomach and the lower part of your esophagus slide up into your chest through the diaphragm. Most people with hiatal hernias have this type.

A paraesophageal hernia is more dangerous. Your esophagus and stomach stay where they should be, but part of your stomach squeezes through the hiatus to sit next to your esophagus. Your stomach can become squeezed and lose its blood supply. Your doctor might call this a strangulated hernia.

BREASKFAST

1. Tuna Casserole

Prep Time: 15 Minutes

Cook Time: 18 Minutes

Servings: 6

Ingredients

- 3 cups egg noodles
- 1 tablespoon butter
- 1 small onion diced
- 2 stalks celery diced
- ⅔ cup frozen peas defrosted
- 1 can tuna 5-6 ounces, drained
- 10 ½ ounces condensed mushroom soup
- ⅓ cup milk
- 1 cup cheddar cheese
- 1 tablespoon parsley

* crumb topping
* ½ cup panko bread crumbs
* 1 tablespoon butter melted
* ½ cup cheddar
* 1 tablespoon parsley

Instructions

1. Preheat oven to 425°F. Combine topping ingredients and set aside.
2. Boil noodles al dente according to package directions. Drain and rinse under cold water.
3. Cook onion and celery in butter until tender, about 5-7 minutes.
4. In a large bowl combine noodles, onion mixture, peas, soup, milk, cheese, tuna and parsley. Mix well.
5. Spread into a 2qt casserole dish and top with crumb topping.
6. Bake 18-20 minutes or until bubbly.

2. Barbecued Hash with Ham and Eggs

Prep Time: 25 Minutes

Cook Time: 45 Minutes

Serves: 4

Ingredients

- 2 tablespoons butter
- ½ small savoy
- cabbage, shredded
- 1 leek, trimmed and diced
- sea salt and ground pepper
- 600 grams cooked new potatoes
- 1 clove garlic, crushed
- 1 teaspoon wholegrain mustard
- 5 tablespoons olive oil
- 4 large eggs
- thin slices ham off the bone or bacon

Instructions

1. Heat the butter over a low heat on a barbecue hotplate. Add the cabbage and leek, season with salt and pepper and fry until golden and soft. Remove from the heat and place in a large bowl. Set aside to cool.

2. Crush the cooked potatoes in your hands and add to the cabbage and leek. Add the garlic and mustard and mix to combine. Season well.

3. Heat 2 tablespoons of the oil over a medium-high heat on the hotplate and using your hands, press the potato mixture into 4 patties. Place on the hotplate and flatten with a spatula. Fry for 3-4 minutes, or until golden and crisp. Carefully flip over and fry for another 3-4 minutes, or until golden.

4. Heat the remaining oil and fry the eggs and as much ham as you like, until cooked to your liking. Serve each patty topped with a fried egg and ham.

3. Crispy Potato Rösti with Hot-Smoked Salmon and Soft Eggs

Prep Time: 15 Minutes

Cook Time: 25 Minutes

Serves: 2

Ingredients

- 700 grams Agria potatoes, scrubbed
- 3 tablespoons melted butter
- 2 cloves garlic, crushed
- 2 teaspoons sea salt
- ground pepper
- 1 tablespoon olive oil

To serve:

- 150 grams hot-smoked salmon
- 2 fried or poached eggs, hot
- your favourite chilli tomato relish or harissa
- purchased dukkah, for sprinkling over

Instructions

1. Grate the potatoes using the large holes on a box grater, trying to get nice long strands. In 2 batches, spread the grated potato out on a large clean tea towel and roll up tightly. Holding the ends, twist like a snake to squeeze out as much liquid as possible, then place the potato in a large bowl. This helps the rösti to get all lovely and crispy. Add the melted butter and garlic and toss with a fork to coat the strands. Season with the salt and a good grind of pepper and toss again.

2. Heat the oil in a non-stick frying pan over a medium heat. Add the potatoes and use a fork to spread into an even layer. Don't press down to compact them. Cover and cook over a medium-low heat for about 10 minutes, or until the base is deeply golden and crisp. Flip the rösti over and cook, uncovered, for another 10 minutes, or until the centre is cooked through.

3. To serve, slide onto a warm plate, top with the salmon and eggs, and dollop a spoonful of chilli tomato relish or harissa on top. Sprinkle with dukkah.

4. Cook's note: You can cook the potatoes as 1
   large rösti or 2 individual serves. Use an 18-
   20cm non-stick pan for 2 individual serves or a
   24-26cm pan for 1.

4. Croque Madame

Prep Time: 10 Minutes

Cook Time: 30 Minutes

Serves: 2

Ingredients

- Béchamel Sauce
- 2 tablespoons butter
- 2 tablespoons plain flour
- 1½ cups whole milk
- 1¼ cups grated parmesan
- pinch freshly grated nutmeg
- 2 teaspoons Dijon mustard
- sea salt and ground pepper
- To Assemble
- 4 large slices sourdough or ciabatta
- 3 tablespoons butter
- 6 slices good-quality ham off the bone
- 1 cup Caramelised Onions (see recipe below, optional)
- ½ cup grated Gruyère cheese

- 2 fried eggs

Instructions

1. Heat the butter in a saucepan over a gentle heat until just melted. Stir in the flour with a wooden spoon. Add the milk in three lots, stirring continuously, until well incorporated. Whisk it while cooking until the sauce is thickened and smooth – it should end up being thick and silky.

2. Add the parmesan, nutmeg and mustard and stir to combine. Season to taste with salt and pepper then refrigerate to cool.

3. Preheat the oven to 200°C regular bake and put an oven tray in to heat.

4. to assemble: Butter one side of each piece of bread. Lay 2 pieces butter-side down on a piece of baking paper. Spread each piece with 3 tablespoons of béchamel sauce and 3 pieces of ham. Top with the onion (if using) and remaining bread, butter side up. Spread with 3 more tablespoons of sauce each. Sprinkle with Gruyère cheese and pop in the oven until

golden and bubbling, for about 15 minutes. Top each sandwich with a fried egg.

Caramelised Onions

Ingredients

- 2 tablespoons olive oil
- 1 tablespoon butter
- 3 large brown onions, sliced 1cm
- 2 cloves garlic, crushed
- 2 teaspoons finely chopped thyme
- sea salt and ground pepper
- 1 tablespoon brown sugar
- 2 tablespoons balsamic vinegar

Instructions

1. Heat the oil and butter in a sauté pan and add the onions, garlic and thyme. Season generously and cook for 20 minutes, stirring occasionally, until softened.
2. Add the sugar and vinegar and continue to cook until deeply golden and glossy.

5. Caramelised Banana and Spiced Whisky Upside-Down Cake

Prep Time: 10 Minutes

Cook Time: 30 Minutes

Serves: 6-8

- Ingredients
  60 grams butter, diced
- ¾ cup brown sugar
- ¼ teaspoon ground cinnamon
- ¼ cup whisky
- 5 medium firm-but-ripe bananas

Cake:

- 1 cup mashed over-ripe bananas (about 3)
- 2 large eggs, size 7
- ½ cup rice bran oil
- ½ cup each brown sugar and caster sugar
- 1 teaspoon vanilla extract
- 2 cups plain flour
- 1 teaspoon baking powder

- ½ teaspoon each ground nutmeg, ground cinnamon, and ground ginger
- ½ teaspoon sea salt

To Serve:

- whipped cream

Instructions

1. Grease a 22cm square x 6cm deep cake tin.
2. Preheat the oven to 160°C fan bake.

Base:

1. Put the butter, sugar and cinnamon in a small saucepan and bring to the boil, stirring to dissolve the sugar. Add the whisky and boil gently for 4 minutes. Cool for 5 minutes then tip into the base of the tin.
2. Slice the bananas lengthways and place cut side down in the tin, trimming them to fit and cover the base. Set aside.

Cake:

1. Whisk the bananas, eggs, oil, both sugars and the vanilla together in a large bowl. Add the

combined flour, baking powder, spices and salt and whisk until well combined. Gently spoon the batter over the bananas, taking care not to dislodge them and smooth the top.

2. Bake for 40 minutes until puffed and golden and a skewer inserted into the centre comes out clean. Leave to cool for 10 minutes then run a knife around the inside of the tin. Invert the cake onto a serving plate with a small rim and replace any bananas that might be stuck on the base along with any caramel.

3. Serve warm or at room temperature with lashings of cream.

6. Brioche Burger

Prep Time: 25 Minutes

Cook Time: 40 Minutes

Serves: 5

Ingredients

- 4-6 large eggs
- 1/3 cup cream
- sea salt and ground pepper
- 20 grams butter
- ¼ cup natural Greek yoghurt
- ¼ cup good-quality egg mayonnaise
- ¼ cup harissa or kasundi

To serve:

- 4 brioche buns, halved and toasted
- 11/3 cups rocket or spinach leaves
- 12 rashers cooked streaky bacon
- 1 avocado, sliced
- 2 tablespoons purchased dukkah

Instructions

1. I'm not sure if this really needs instructions but here we go! Whisk the eggs and cream together and season with salt and pepper. Heat the butter over a gentle heat in a frying pan and add the eggs. Don't stir for about 30 seconds, then cook, stirring only occasionally, until the eggs are softly set.
2. Whisk the yoghurt and mayonnaise together and swirl through the harissa or kasundi.
3. Serve the buns slathered in the spicy yoghurt mix and topped with rocket, bacon, avocado and egg, and finished with a sprinkling of dukkah.

7. Sweetcorn Fritters with Smashed Avocado

Prep Time: 25 Minutes

Cook Time: 40 Minutes

Serves: 5

Ingredients

- ½ cup plain flour
- ½ teaspoon baking powder
- 1 teaspoon each sea salt, smoked paprika and cumin seeds
- ¼ cup chopped coriander, plus extra to garnish
- 1 large egg, size 7
- 2–3 tablespoons milk
- 1½ cups corn kernels (or kernels from 2 large corn cobs)
- olive oil for cooking

To Serve:

- Smashed Avocado

- Sour Cream Dressing
- Smashed Avocado:
- 2 large, ripe avocados
- 2–3 tablespoons lime juice
- 2 tablespoons finely
- chopped coriander
- sea salt and ground pepper
- Sour Cream Dressing:
- ½ cup each sour cream and thick plain yoghurt
- 2 cloves garlic, crushed
- finely grated zest 1 lime
- 1 tablespoon lime juice
- sea salt and ground pepper

Instructions

1. Put all the dry ingredients, along with the coriander, in a large bowl and combine.
2. Whisk the egg and 2 tablespoons of milk together, then stir into the dry ingredients until well mixed. Add the corn and, if the mixture is really thick, stir in the remaining milk.

3. Heat a little oil in a sauté pan and cook spoonfuls of the mixture over a medium heat for about 3 minutes until cooked through. Drain on kitchen towels and keep warm in a low oven.
4. Divide the fritters among plates. Top with the smashed avocado, sour cream dressing and extra coriander.
5. Smashed Avocado:
6. Roughly crush the avocado flesh with a fork then stir in the remaining ingredients. Season generously.
7. Makes about 1½ cups
8. Sour Cream Dressing:
9. Whisk the sour cream until smooth, then stir in the remaining ingredients and season well. Cover and chill until ready to serve.

Makes 1 cup

8. Boozy Barbecued Stone Fruit Parcels

Prep Time: 35 Minutes

Cook Time: 50 Minutes

Serves: 3

Ingredients

Fruit:

- 1 peach
- 1 nectarine
- 2 apricots
- 2 plums

Parcels:

- 3 gingernut biscuits, roughly broken
- 1 tablespoon whisky (or use your own favourite tipple)
- 1-2 tablespoons honey, depending on the ripeness of the fruit
- 1 teaspoon orange zest
- 1 tablespoon orange juice

- 1/3 piece vanilla bean, split with seeds scraped out or use ¼ teaspoon vanilla extract
- 2 teaspoons butter

Instructions

11. Cut out a 20cm x 20cm piece each of baking paper and foil.
12. FRUIT: Halve and stone the fruit, cutting any larger pieces into quarters.
13. PARCELS: Place the baking paper over the foil and scatter over the biscuits. Arrange the fruit over the biscuits. Stir together the whisky, honey, zest and juice and vanilla bean seeds or extract and pour over the fruit. Nestle in the vanilla bean and dot over the butter. Bring the sides together and fold to seal tightly. Place on a heated barbecue and cook for 15-20 minutes, or until the fruit is tender.
14. TO SERVE: Open the parcel and serve with a scoop of ice cream, runny cream or yoghurt.
15. Makes 1 generous parcel

9. Spiced Cauliflower Rice Bowls with Soft Eggs And Chutney

Prep Time: 35 Minutes

Cook Time: 50 Minutes

Serves: 3

Ingredients

- 1 small cauliflower, cut into quarters
- 2 tablespoons olive oil
- good knob of butter
- 3 spring onions, thinly sliced
- 2 cloves garlic, crushed
- 2 teaspoons mild curry powder
- 1 teaspoon each ground cumin and ground ginger
- ¼ teaspoon ground turmeric
- ¼ – ½ teaspoon chilli flakes
- sea salt and ground pepper
- small handful coriander, chopped, plus extra for garnish

- To Serve:
- 2 eggs, either soft-boiled and halved, poached or fried
- thick plain yoghurt, mango or tamarind chutney, toasted sesame seeds and chilli flakes

Instructions

1. Grate the cauliflower on the coarse side of a box grater, discarding the tough stem. It looks a lot but reduces when cooked.
2. Heat a wide sauté pan with the oil and butter. When hot, add the spring onion, garlic and all the spices and cook for 2 minutes.
3. Add the cauliflower and season generously with salt and pepper. Cook over a high heat for 3-5 minutes, or until the cauliflower is only just tender but still has a bite to it, stirring often so it's all coated in the spices. Fold through the coriander.
4. TO SERVE: Divide the spiced cauliflower between bowls and top with yoghurt, chutney and the eggs. Garnish with sesame seeds, chilli and more coriander.

5. COOK'S NOTE: Top with slices of grilled haloumi, crispy bacon, hot smoked salmon or wedges of roasted pumpkin.

10. Fluffy Buttermilk Hotcakes

Prep Time: 35 Minutes

Cook Time: 50 Minutes

Serves: 3

Ingredients

- 1 cup plain flour
- 3 tablespoons caster sugar
- 1 teaspoon baking powder
- ½ teaspoon baking soda
- ½ teaspoon salt
- ¾ cup buttermilk
- 2 tablespoons melted butter
- 1 teaspoon vanilla extract
- 1 large egg, separated
- extra butter for cooking

Instructions

1. Combine all the dry ingredients in a large bowl.

2. Whisk the buttermilk, melted butter, vanilla extract and the egg yolk together.

3. In another bowl, whisk the egg white to firmish peaks.

4. Add the wet ingredients to the dry ingredients and stir to combine. Gently but thoroughly fold in the egg white, keeping as much air in the batter as possible.

5. To cook: Heat a knob of butter in a large non-stick sauté pan over a medium heat. Add ¼ cups of batter and cook until small holes appear in the surface. Turn over and cook for 1-2 minutes, or until puffed and golden and they feel firm to the touch.

6. Keep the hotcakes warm in a low oven on a cooling rack and repeat with the remaining batter.

7. Makes 6 medium hotcakes

8. Additions To Batter:

9. Blueberries and a pinch of cinnamon

10. Raspberries and a pinch of nutmeg

11. Lemon zest

12. Serving Suggestions:

13. Maple syrup, golden syrup or honey

14. Crispy bacon, sliced bananas, fresh berries, sliced stone fruit, roasted apples or pears, yoghurt, crème fraîche, sour cream, mascarpone

11. Chipotle Lime and Garlic Squid

Prep Time: 15 Minutes

Cook Time: 55 Minutes

Serves: 5

Ingredients

Squid:

- 500 grams frozen squid tubes
- ½ cup plain flour
- ½ cup semolina flour
- ⅓ cup fine polenta
- 2 teaspoons garlic powder
- 2 teaspoons chipotle powder
- 1 teaspoon table salt
- vegetable oil, for frying
- 2 cloves garlic, finely sliced
- 1 red chilli, sliced
- olive oil

- finely grated zest ½ lime, plus juice to serve
- sea salt
- good-quality egg mayonnaise, to serve

Instructions

1. Defrost and rinse the squid tubes, then cut into shapes. I like to do a combination of rings and lattice-scored rectangles.
2. In a large bowl, combine the flours, polenta, garlic powder, chipotle powder and salt.
3. Heat 5cm of vegetable oil to 180°C in a large saucepan. Dredge the squid in the flour mixture and fry in batches until golden and crisp. Remove with a slotted spoon and drain on a tray lined with paper towels.
4. In a small frying pan, briefly fry the garlic and chilli in a little olive oil until the garlic is just starting to colour.
5. In a large bowl, toss together the squid, lime zest, fried garlic and chilli and sea salt to taste.
6. Serve hot with mayonnaise and a squeeze of lime juice.

12. Petra Shawarma's Babaghanoush

Prep Time: 30 Minutes

Cook Time: 40 Minutes

Serves: 4

Ingredients

- 3 medium eggplants
- 4 tablespoons extra-virgin olive oil, plus extra to serve
- 2 cloves garlic
- 1 tablespoon best-quality tahini
- zest ½ lemon
- juice 2 lemons
- sea salt and ground pepper, to taste
- sumac, to sprinkle over
- small handful curly parsley, finely chopped
- ½ small tomato, deseeded and chopped, optional

Instructions

1. Preheat the oven to 180°C.
2. Cut the eggplants in half lengthways and toss with 2 tablespoons of the olive oil. Arrange on a baking tray, flesh side up, and bake for around 45 minutes, or until soft. Remove the eggplant from the oven and set aside to cool. Once cool, scoop out of the flesh and set aside. Peel and grate the garlic into a medium-sized bowl. Add the tahini, remaining 2 tablespoons olive oil, eggplant, lemon zest and lemon juice to the bowl. Use a whisk or spatula to combine all the ingredients and season with salt and pepper to taste. Transfer to a serving bowl, sprinkle with sumac and parsley, top with tomato, if using, and drizzle with extra olive oil.
3. Cook's note: You can also grill the eggplant on the stove or a barbecue grill instead of baking it.

13. Roast Salmon with Tahini Yoghurt Mayo

Prep Time: 15 Minutes

Cook Time: 35 Minutes

Serves: 6-8

Ingredients

Salmon:

- 1.5-kilogram (approx) side of salmon
- 2 tablespoons extra-virgin olive oil
- 4 cloves garlic, crushed
- 2 tablespoons pomegranate molasses
- 1 teaspoon cumin seeds
- 1 teaspoon sumac
- 1 teaspoon sea salt

Tahini Yoghurt Mayo

- 1 cup thick plain yoghurt
- ¼ cup good-quality egg mayonnaise
- ¼ cup tahini

- finely grated zest 1 lemon
- 1 clove garlic, crushed
- 1 teaspoon each ground cumin and sea salt
- Pickled Red Onions
- ¼ cup cider vinegar
- 2 teaspoons caster sugar
- ½ teaspoon sea salt
- 1 small red onion, thinly sliced

To Serve

- ⅔ cup chopped walnuts, toasted
- 1/3 cup each fresh coriander and mint leaves

Instructions

1. Preheat the oven to 220°C fan bake.
2. Salmon: Lay the salmon skin side down on the lined oven tray. Combine the olive oil, garlic, pomegranate molasses, cumin seeds, sumac and salt. Brush over the salmon and bake for 12 minutes. Take care to not overcook it.
3. Tahini Yoghurt Mayo: Whisk all the ingredients together until smooth and creamy.

4. Pickled Red Onions: Put the vinegar, sugar and salt in a small non-reactive bowl and whisk to dissolve the sugar. Add the onion, cover and refrigerate until ready to use.

5. To Serve: When ready to serve, garnish the salmon with the drained onion, walnuts and herbs. Serve with the Tahini Yoghurt Mayo.

14. Spag Bol Mince and Cheese Pie

Prep Time: 20 Minutes

Cook Time: 45 Minutes

Serves: 8-10

Ingredients

- 2 tablespoons olive oil
- 120 grams pancetta or streaky bacon, chopped
- 1 onion, finely chopped
- 1 stick celery, finely chopped
- 1 carrot, finely chopped
- ⅛-¼ teaspoon chilli flakes, to taste
- sea salt and ground pepper
- 4 cloves garlic, crushed
- 500 grams beef mince
- 500 grams pork mince
- ¼ cup milk
- ¼ teaspoon freshly grated nutmeg
- 1 cup red wine
- 2 tablespoons tomato paste
- 1 teaspoon caster sugar

- 2 x 400-gram tins chopped tomatoes
- 1½ cups grated colby
- 800 grams good-quality puff pastry (I used Paneton)
- 1 large egg yolk whisked with
- 1 tablespoon milk or cream

To serve

- good-quality purchased tomato chutney
- Equipment: Grease a 24cm x 34cm foil roasting dish.

Instructions

1. Heat the olive oil in a large heavy-based saucepan. Add the pancetta and cook over a medium heat for 3-4 minutes, until crispy. Add the onion, celery, carrot and chilli flakes. Season with salt and pepper and cook for a further 10 minutes, stirring.
2. Add the garlic and both minces, using a fork to break up the meat as it cooks. Cook for 5-8 minutes until the meat is no longer pink.

3. Add the ¼ cup milk and nutmeg and cook for 5 minutes, then stir through the red wine, tomato paste, sugar and tomatoes. Cook, half-covered over a low heat, for 3 hours, then remove the lid and cook for a further 45 minutes, until most of the liquid has been absorbed. It only needs to be stirred every half hour. Chill for at least 1 hour.

4. Preheat the oven to 180°C fan bake.

5. Line the greased roasting dish with pastry – reserving enough to use as the pie 'lid' and for decoration if desired. Put the filling into the pastry-lined tin. Whisk the egg and 1 tablespoon milk or cream and brush a little around the exposed pastry edge. Top with remaining pastry cut to fit. Crimp the edges, sealing with the tines of a fork. Brush with remaining egg and decorate if desired with cut out pastry shapes. Bake for 40 minutes, until golden. Snip the foil tin away from the pie to remove it and serve with tomato chutney.

15. Moroccan Baked Chicken with Pearl Couscous

Prep Time: 20 Minutes

Cook Time: 45 Minutes

Serves: 4-6

Ingredients

- 6 chicken drumsticks
- 4-5 bone-in, skin-on chicken thighs
- sea salt and ground pepper
- 2 tablespoons olive oil
- 2 brown onions, peeled, cut into quarters through the root
- 2 tablespoons honey
- 2 tablespoons tomato paste
- zest and juice 1 lemon
- 3 tablespoons purchased Moroccan spice mix (I use Simon Gault's)
- 3 cloves garlic, crushed
- 1½ cups pearl couscous (also called mograbieh)

- 3¾ cups chicken stock
- 3 bay leaves
- 1 cinnamon stick
- 12 green or black olives

To serve

- 2 tablespoons finely chopped pistachios
- 2 tablespoons finely chopped parsley
- Equipment: Large roasting dish or ovenproof baking dish big enough to take everything in a single layer (my tray is 42cm x 32cm x 3cm deep).

Instruction

1. Preheat the oven to 180°C fan bake.
2. Season the chicken with salt and pepper. Heat the oil in a large frying pan and cook the chicken skin side down until deeply golden brown. Transfer to the roasting dish. Don't wash the pan.
3. Add the onions to the pan and cook for 5 minutes, then add to the chicken. In a small bowl, stir the honey, tomato paste, lemon zest

and juice, spice mix and garlic together, then tip into the pan and cook for 2 minutes. Stir in the couscous, stock, bay leaves and the cinnamon stick and bring to the boil.

4. Tip the mixture over the chicken and onions then distribute the couscous evenly so it's not all clumped together and flick off any that's on top of the chicken.

5. Cover tightly with foil and bake for 25 minutes. Uncover, scatter over the olives, then bake for a further 15 minutes, or until the chicken is fully cooked and the couscous is tender but still with a little bite. Scatter over the combined pistachios and parsley.

16. Spice Sweet

Prep Time: 34 Minutes

Cook Time: 55 Minutes

Serves: 4

Ingredients

- ½ cup plain flour
- sea salt and ground pepper
- 750 grams grass-fed slow-cook venison, diced
- 2 tablespoons rice bran oil
- 2 large onions, thinly sliced
- 3 cloves garlic, crushed
- 1 tablespoon grated fresh ginger
- ¼ cup oyster sauce
- ¼ cup sweet chilli sauce
- 2 tablespoons soy sauce
- 2 whole star anise
- 2 cinnamon sticks
- ½ cup beef stock
- ½ cup coconut cream

- 12 fresh shiitake mushrooms, stems trimmed, or use small portobello mushrooms

To serve

- ½ cup crispy roasted shallots

Instructions

1. Preheat the oven to 130°C regular bake.
2. Put the flour in a large bowl and season well with salt and pepper. Toss the venison in the flour, shaking off the excess. Heat the oil in a large frying pan and brown the venison in batches. Use a slotted spoon to transfer to a medium casserole dish. Don't let the flour catch and burn, and add more oil to the pan as needed.
3. Add the onions to the frying pan with a good pinch of salt. Cover and cook for 8 minutes, stirring occasionally and adding a splash of water if the pan is too dry.
4. Stir in the garlic, ginger, oyster sauce, sweet chilli sauce, soy sauce, star anise and cinnamon sticks and bring to the boil, scraping the base

of the pan to release any sticky bits. Add the beef stock and coconut cream and bring to the boil. Return the meat and any juices to the pan and combine. Cover tightly with a lid. Braise for 2 hours, then add the mushrooms to the pan, pushing them down into the sauce. Cover and continue to cook for 1 hour, or until the meat is very tender.

5. Serve with steamed Asian greens and hot cooked rice.

17. Smoky Chipotle Braised Venison

Prep Time: 15 Minutes

Cook Time: 45 Minutes

Serves: 4-6

Ingredients

* 1 kilogram diced venison
* sea salt and ground pepper
* 2 tablespoons olive oil
* 3 brown onions, thinly sliced
* 2 bay leaves
* 3 cloves garlic, crushed
* 2 teaspoons each dried oregano, ground cumin and smoked paprika
* ½ teaspoon ground cinnamon
* sea salt and ground pepper
* 1 tablespoon each sherry vinegar or red wine vinegar and brown sugar
* 2 whole chipotle peppers in adobo sauce, roughly chopped

- 2 tablespoons each tomato paste, wholegrain mustard, adobo sauce from the peppers and plain flour
- ½ cup red wine
- ¾ cup good-quality beef stock

Crispy Garlicky Crumbs:

- 3 tablespoons olive oil
- 1 tablespoon butter
- 1½ cups fresh sourdough breadcrumbs
- 2 cloves garlic, crushed
- 2 tablespoons finely
- chopped parsley

Instruction

1. Preheat the oven to 120°C regular bake.
2. Trim any silverskin off the venison and season with salt and pepper. Set aside.
3. Heat the oil in an ovenproof casserole dish and add the onions, bay leaves, garlic, oregano and spices with a splash of water. Add a good pinch of salt, cover and cook for 10 minutes over a medium-low heat, stirring often and adding a

splash more water if needed. (The water will evaporate off.) Combine the vinegar, sugar, chipotle peppers, tomato paste, mustard, adobo sauce and flour in a bowl, then stir in the wine. Add to the onions and cook for 3 minutes. Add the stock, season and bring to the boil. Add the seasoned venison to the pot, stir to combine and heat until it just comes to the boil. Press a circle of baking paper down onto the meat then cover the dish tightly with a lid or foil. Place in the oven and cook for 50 minutes, stirring after 30 minutes.

4. CRUMBS: Heat the oil and butter in a large frying pan and cook the crumbs until golden and crisp, stirring often. Stir in the garlic and parsley and season well. Scatter over the venison when serving.

5. Cook's note: We served the venison with mashed potatoes and flash-fried green beans.

18. Indonesian-Style Coconut and Lamb Shank Curry

Prep Time: 25 Minutes

Cook Time: 50 Minutes

Serves: 4

Ingredients

Paste:

- 2 lemongrass stalks, tough outer skin removed, finely chopped
- 3cm piece ginger, chopped
- 5 cloves garlic
- 2 red chillies

Curry:

- 2 tablespoons neutral oil
- 4 lamb shanks, roughly 1.5 kilograms
- 6 shallots, halved
- 6 cardamom pods, toasted
- 1 teaspoon each ground cumin and coriander

- ½ teaspoon ground turmeric
- 2 cups chicken stock
- 400ml tin coconut cream
- 1 makrut lime leaf
- 2 cinnamon sticks
- 2 star anise
- 1 tablespoon each tamarind paste and brown sugar
- 1 teaspoon sea salt
- 2 dried red chillies
- 80 grams desiccated coconut
- 1 tablespoon each lime juice and brown sugar

Instructions

1. Preheat the oven to 160°C regular bake.
2. PASTE: Blitz all the ingredients in a food processor.
3. CURRY: In a large ovenproof casserole dish, heat the oil over a medium heat. Brown the shanks on all sides, then set aside. Reduce the heat to low, add the paste the pan and fry for 3 minutes, stirring regularly. Add the shallots, cardamom pods and ground spices and fry for a

further 2 minutes. Add the lamb, stock, coconut cream, lime leaf, cinnamon, star anise, tamarind, brown sugar, sea salt and chillies and bring to a simmer. Cover and cook in the oven for 3 hours, or until the meat is tender. Toast the coconut in a frying pan over a medium heat until golden, then set aside. Remove the lamb from the curry, set aside and cover with foil. Increase the oven to 180°C regular bake. Add the coconut, lime juice and sugar to the curry and season with salt. Return to the oven for 15 minutes, uncovered. Once thickened, return the shanks to the curry and return to the oven briefly to warm through.

19. Braised Nutty Satay Chicken

Prep Time: 15 Minutes

Cook Time: 50 Minutes

Serves: 4

Ingredients

- 1½ teaspoons each ground cumin, coriander, turmeric, chilli powder, curry powder and sea salt
- 8 skinless, boneless chicken thighs
- 2 tablespoons olive oil
- 400ml tin coconut cream
- ½ cup each chicken stock and peanut butter
- 2 tablespoons kecap manis
- 1 tablespoon brown sugar
- 1 tablespoon rice wine vinegar
- finely grated zest and juice 1 large lime
- 1 teaspoon sesame oil
- 3 cloves garlic, crushed
- 1 tablespoon grated fresh ginger
- 4 small whole red chillies

- 1 stalk lemongrass, lightly bruised with a rolling pin
- ½ cup roasted peanuts, to garnish

Instructions

1. Preheat the oven to 180°C fan bake.
2. Combine all the spices and salt in a large bowl. Add the chicken and toss so each piece is well coated. Heat the oil in a large ovenproof frying pan over a medium heat and quickly brown the chicken on both sides. Transfer to a plate. Combine all the remaining ingredients except the chillies, lemongrass and peanuts in a large bowl. Tip into the frying pan and bring to the boil, crushing the peanut butter with a fork to amalgamate. Add the chicken and juices to the pan and turn to coat in the sauce. Nestle in the chillies and lemongrass. Bake for 35-40 minutes, or until the chicken is fully cooked. Top with the peanuts to serve.

20. Stir-Fried Beef with Green Beans, Gochujang and Kimchi

Prep Time: 20 Minutes

Cook Time: 55 Minutes

Serves: 2

Ingredients

Sauce:

- 3 tablespoons gochujang (Korean red pepper paste)
- 2 tablespoons honey
- 1 tablespoon soy sauce
- 1 tablespoon grated fresh ginger
- 2 cloves garlic, crushed
- 2 teaspoons sesame oil
- 2 teaspoons rice vinegar
- ½-1 teaspoon chilli flakes, to taste

To cook and serve:

- 300 grams beef schnitzel, sliced into very thin strips
- sea salt and ground pepper
- vegetable oil
- 200 grams slim green beans, thinly sliced on the diagonal
- 1½ cups kimchi
- toasted sesame seeds and finely chopped coriander, to serve
- hot cooked noodles or rice, to serve

Instructions

1. Sauce: Mix all the ingredients together and set aside.
2. To cook and serve: Season the steak with salt and pepper. Heat a large frying pan with a little oil until searing hot. Add the steak in small batches and cook for 10-15 seconds. Transfer to a plate and cover to keep warm while you cook the remaining steak. Add a little more oil to the pan, add the beans and cook until lightly blistered. Add the kimchi and cook for 2 minutes, tossing together. Tip in the sauce and

let it bubble up. Add the beef and resting juices and stir everything together.

3. Divide between bowls and top with the sesame seeds and coriander. Serve with noodles or rice.

4. Cook's note: The steak needs to be wafer-thin so it will cook in seconds and remain tender. Place the schnitzel between 2 pieces of plastic wrap and flatten with a rolling pin before cutting into 2cm-wide strips.

21. Lemon Roast Chicken with Pistachio And Green Olive Dressing

Prep Time: 25 Minutes

Cook Time: 55 Minutes

Serves: 4

Ingredients

- 1 kilogram Agria potatoes, peeled and sliced 1cm thick
- 1 large brown onion, thinly sliced
- 400-gram tin crushed Italian tomatoes
- ½ cup white wine
- 2 cloves garlic, crushed
- sea salt and ground pepper
- 1 Rangitikei Free Range whole chicken
- 1 large lemon, halved
- bunch woody herbs, use any combination of rosemary, thyme and bay leaves

- 1 tablespoon olive oil
- Olive and Pistachio Dressing
- ½ cup roughly chopped green olives
- ¼ cup pistachios, chopped
- ¼ cup each mint and parsley leaves, finely chopped
- 2 cloves garlic, crushed
- 2 teaspoons finely grated lemon zest
- 1 tablespoon lemon juice
- 1/3 cup olive oil
- ½-1 teaspoon honey, to taste

Instructions

1. Preheat the oven to 170°C fan bake. Toss the potatoes, onion, tomatoes, wine and garlic in a large bowl and season. Spread evenly in a roasting dish and bake for 30 minutes.
2. Season the chicken cavity and squeeze in the lemon, then add the squeezed halves and herbs. Tie the legs with kitchen string and tuck the wings under. Place on top of the potatoes. Brush with oil and season well. Roast for 1½

hours, or until fully cooked.

3. Dressing: Combine all the ingredients and season well.

4. To serve: Spoon over some dressing, serving the rest separately.

22. Three-Cheese Mac'n'pork Meatballs

Prep Time: 30 Minutes

Cook Time: 50 Minutes

Serves: 6

Ingredients

Meatballs:

- 1/3 cup panko breadcrumbs
- 150 grams ricotta or cottage cheese
- ½ cup freshly grated parmesan
- 2 tablespoons milk or water
- 1 large egg
- 1 tablespoon dried oregano
- 2 cloves garlic, crushed
- 1 teaspoon sea salt
- finely grated zest 1 lemon
- 500 grams pork mince

To cook:

- 1 tablespoon each olive oil and butter
- 1 onion, thinly sliced

- 1 leek, thinly sliced
- 3 cloves garlic, crushed
- 2 teaspoons fennel seeds
- ¼-½ teaspoon chilli flakes
- sea salt and ground pepper
- 50 grams butter
- ¼ cup plain flour
- 3 cups whole milk
- ½ cup cream
- 2 teaspoons Dijon mustard
- ½ teaspoon grated nutmeg
- 100 grams cheddar, grated, plus 30 grams extra for topping
- 60 grams gruyère, grated, plus 30 grams extra for topping
- ½ cup freshly grated parmesan, plus ½ cup extra for topping
- 500 grams macaroni or other small tube pasta
- Equipment: 6-cup capacity ovenproof baking dish.

Instructions

6. Preheat the oven to 180°C fan bake.

7. Meatballs: Combine all the ingredients except the pork in a large bowl and leave for 15 minutes. Add the pork and mix until fully combined. Hands are good for this. Form into about 24 large walnut-sized meatballs. Heat a little oil in a large frying pan and, when hot, quickly brown the meatballs. They won't be fully cooked. Set aside. The meatballs can be browned several hours ahead of assembling.

8. To cook: Heat the oil and butter in a large frying pan and cook the onion, leek, garlic, fennel seeds and chilli with a good pinch of salt for 10 minutes or until very tender. Set aside.

9. Melt the 50 grams butter in a large saucepan and whisk in the flour until smooth. Cook over a low heat for 1 minute, then gradually whisk in the combined milk and cream, whisking continuously until smooth. Stir in the mustard and nutmeg and season well. Simmer for 5 minutes, stirring often. Remove from the heat and stir in the three cheeses until melted and

smooth. Stir in three-quarters of the leek mixture and set the rest aside.

Cook the pasta in plenty of salted boiling water for 2 minutes less than the package instructions, then drain well. Combine the pasta with the sauce and tip into the baking dish. Nestle in the meatballs, then dot over the remaining leek mixture. Scatter over the combined leftover three cheeses and bake for 25 minutes, until golden and bubbling around the edges.

23. Crispy Fried Soy and Ginger Chicken Bao

Prep Time: 15 Minutes

Cook Time: 45 Minutes

Serves: 6

Ingredients

Chicken:

- 330 grams Rangitikei Free Range skinless boneless chicken thighs
- 2 tablespoons soy sauce
- 1 tablespoon grated fresh ginger
- 2 teaspoons gochujang chilli paste or other chilli paste
- 1 teaspoon sesame oil
- 3 cloves garlic, crushed
- 1 cup potato flour
- sea salt and ground pepper
- vegetable oil for cooking

To Serve:

- good-quality egg mayonnaise
- gochujang or other chilli sauce
- 6 bao buns, steamed and warm
- pickled chillies
- Quick Pickled Red Onion
- coriander

Instructions

1. Cut the chicken into bite-size pieces. Place in a large bowl with all the remaining ingredients and mix well. Cover and chill for 2-24 hours. Remove from the fridge 1 hour before cooking.
2. Heat 4cm of oil in a wok or a deep, medium-sized saucepan until a small piece of bread dropped in turns golden in 30 seconds.
3. Put the potato flour in a bowl and season well. Drain the chicken, then coat in flour, shaking off the excess. Cook for about 2 minutes each side until golden and fully cooked. Drain on a rack set over a baking tray in a warm oven until all the chicken is cooked.
4. To serve: Marble a little mayo and gochujang or other chilli sauce together and spread on both

sides of the buns. Fill with the chicken, pickled chillies, Quick Pickled Red Onion and coriander and serve immediately.

5. Quick Pickled Red Onion

Ingredients

- ½ teaspoon sea salt
- ½ teaspoon caster sugar
- 1 medium red onion, very thinly sliced
- 2 tablespoons apple cider vinegar

Method

1. Combine all the ingredients in a small bowl. Leave for 30 minutes, turning occasionally. Drain before using. Onions will keep for 1 week in the fridge.

24. Three-Cheese and Pumpkin Baked Pasta

Prep Time: 20 Minutes

Cook Time: 60 Minutes

Serves: 6-8

Ingredients

- 1½ kilograms butternut or crown pumpkin, peeled and seeded
- olive oil
- sea salt and ground pepper
- 500 grams medium pasta tubes, e.g., penne or rigatoni
- 4 packed cups spinach leaves, well washed and roughly ripped
- 1 tablespoon olive oil
- 2 tablespoons tomato purée
- 3 cloves garlic, crushed
- 1 teaspoon sea salt

- ½ teaspoon each ground black pepper and chilli flakes
- 1 teaspoon freshly grated nutmeg
- 1 cup cream
- 1 cup each grated parmesan, gruyère and mozzarella
- 125-gram ball fresh mozzarella in whey, drained
- ¼ cup chopped pine nuts
- Equipment: 24cm x 30cm ovenproof baking dish.

Instructions

2. Preheat the oven to 180°C fan bake.
3. Cut the pumpkin into bite-sized chunks and place on a large baking tray. Toss with olive oil and season with salt and pepper. Cover with foil and roast until tender, about 30 minutes. Set aside.
4. Cook the pasta in a large pot of boiling salted water according to the packet instructions, adding the spinach for the last 30 seconds.

Drain the pasta and spinach well, then toss with the oil. Set aside.

5. Put half the roasted pumpkin into a food processor along with the tomato purée, garlic, salt, pepper, chilli, nutmeg and cream. Blend briefly until smooth. Tip into a large bowl and stir in ¾ cup each of the three grated cheeses and the remaining pumpkin. Add the pasta and spinach and combine.

6. Tip into the baking dish, then break over the fresh mozzarella and sprinkle with the remaining grated cheese and the pine nuts. Season with salt and pepper. Bake for 25 minutes, until golden and bubbling.

25. Chicken Scallopine With Artichokes, Pappardelle and Lemon Crème Fraîche

Prep Time: 30 Minutes

Cook Time: 55 Minutes

Serves: 6

Ingredients

- ½ cup plain flour
- sea salt and ground pepper
- 600 grams skinless, boneless Rangitikei chicken breasts, cut thinly on an angle into ½ cm-thick slices
- 2 tablespoons each olive oil and butter
- 340-gram jar artichoke quarters, drained
- 1 cup white wine
- 3 tablespoons capers, well drained
- 2 cloves garlic, crushed
- finely grated zest 1 lemon
- pinch chilli flakes
- 2 packed cups baby spinach leaves

- 200 grams crème fraîche
- 250 grams pappardelle, cooked and hot
- 2 tablespoons parsley, finely chopped

Instructions

1. Season the flour and coat the chicken, shaking off the excess flour.
2. Heat half the oil and butter in a large frying pan and fry the chicken in batches until cooked through, adding the remaining oil and butter between batches. Transfer to a plate and cover to keep warm.
3. Add the artichokes, wine, capers, garlic, zest and chilli flakes to the pan and let it bubble up and reduce a little. Add the spinach, turning to wilt. Season, then stir in the crème fraîche until melted and bubbling. Add the chicken with the resting juices, then stir in the pasta, turning to combine. Add the parsley and serve in warm shallow bowls.

26. Yellow Curry Lentil Soup

Prep Time: 20 Minutes

Cook Time: 50 Minutes

Serves: 4

Ingredients

- 2 tablespoons olive oil
- 1 onion, chopped
- 3 garlic cloves, crushed
- 1 tablespoon grated fresh ginger
- 2 teaspoons fish sauce
- ½ cup Thai yellow curry paste
- 3 cups good-quality chicken or vegetable stock
- 400ml coconut milk
- 2 makrut lime leaves
- 1 large kūmara, peeled and chopped
- 400-gram tin black or brown lentils, drained
- 200 grams green beans, trimmed and halved

To serve

- 1/3 cup roughly chopped roasted cashews

Instructions

1. Heat the oil in a large pot or deep frying pan and add the onion. Cook over a medium heat for 8 minutes, until softened but not coloured. Add the garlic, ginger, fish sauce and curry paste and stir to combine. Add the stock, coconut milk and lime leaves and bring to a simmer for 5 minutes. Add the kūmara and cook for a further 15 minutes, or until just cooked through. Add the lentils and beans, cook for a final 5 minutes, then serve immediately.

27. Garlic Mashed Potatoes with Crunchy Seedy Crumbs

Prep Time: 35 Minutes

Cook Time: 50 Minutes

Serves: 6

Ingredients

- 1½ kilograms Agria potatoes
- 1 cup cream
- ½ cup milk
- 2 cloves garlic, crushed
- 50 grams butter
- sea salt and ground pepper

To Serve:

- Crunchy Seedy Crumbs (see recipe below)
- extra butter, optional

Instructions

1. Peel the potatoes and cut into large chunks. Cook in a large saucepan of well-salted boiling water until tender. Drain well and return to the saucepan. Place back over a low heat for a couple of minutes to drive off excess water. Heat the cream, milk and garlic in a microwave or small saucepan. Mash the potatoes until smooth or push through a potato ricer, then stir in the hot cream mixture and the butter until smooth. Season well. Transfer to a serving bowl and top with a couple of spoonfuls of the Crunchy Seedy Crumbs and another knob of butter, if desired. Serve the remaining crumbs alongside.
2. Crunchy Seedy Crumbs

Ingredients

- 1 cup pumpkin seeds
- ½ cup sunflower seeds
- 2 tablespoons sesame seeds
- 2 tablespoons maple syrup
- 2 tablespoons olive oil
- 2 teaspoons smoked paprika

- 1 teaspoon chilli flakes
- sea salt

Instructions

1. Combine everything except the salt in a large bowl and toss to coat well. Tip into a large frying pan over a low heat and cook, stirring occasionally, until golden and fragrant. Season generously with sea salt. Tip onto a large plate and, when cool, transfer to an airtight container.

28. Lisa's Spice-Baked Chicken with Autumn Veges And Lentils

Prep Time: 20 Minutes

Cook Time: 45 Minutes

Serves: 4

Ingredients

- 2 tablespoons each olive oil, maple syrup, soy sauce and apple cider vinegar
- 2 teaspoons each ground cumin and smoked paprika
- 1 teaspoon ground turmeric
- ½ teaspoon chilli flakes
- 3 cloves garlic, crushed
- 1 x 400-gram tin each brown lentils, drained and rinsed, and cherry tomatoes
- 6 chicken thighs, skin on, bone in
- 2 red onions, cut into quarters through the root
- 1 eggplant, halved lengthways and each half cut into 4 large chunks

- ½ medium butternut pumpkin, cut into 1½ cm-thick slices, skin on
- sea salt and ground pepper

To Serve:

- Garlicky Lemon Spinach (see recipe below)
- 1 cup thick plain yoghurt
- chilli flakes
- Equipment: Large, shallow roasting tray, at least 40cm x 26cm.

Instructions

1. Preheat the oven to 170°C fan bake.
2. Combine all the ingredients down to and including the lentils and tomatoes in a large bowl. Add the chicken and vegetables and turn to coat well. Tip onto the tray and spread into a single layer. Season and bake for 30 minutes. Turn the vegetables over and baste the chicken. Cook for a further 15-20 minutes, or until the chicken is fully cooked. Top with the spinach, a dollop of yoghurt and sprinkle of chilli flakes.
3. Garlicky Lemon Spinach

Ingredients

- 2 tablespoons olive oil
- 2 cloves garlic, crushed
- finely grated zest 1 lemon
- 3 tightly packed cups baby spinach leaves
- 1 tablespoon lemon juice
- sea salt and ground pepper

Instructions

1. Heat the oil in a large frying pan over a medium heat. Sizzle the garlic and zest for about 30 seconds. Add the spinach and turn to lightly wilt, then add the juice. This should take under 1 minute. Tip into a bowl and season.

29. Braised Chicken with Bacon, Mushrooms And Fennel

Prep Time: 15 Minutes

Cook Time: 45 Minutes

Serves: 6

Ingredients

- 1 tablespoon olive oil
- knob of butter
- 2 whole chicken legs (leg and thigh)
- sea salt and ground pepper
- 100 grams streaky bacon, sliced into 2cm pieces
- 1 leek, thickly sliced
- 1 fennel bulb, cut into thick wedges through the root
- 2 bay leaves
- 2 cloves garlic, crushed
- 2 teaspoons finely chopped rosemary

- 250 grams medium Portobello mushrooms, halved
- ½ cup Marsala wine or white wine
- ½ cup chicken stock
- Equipment: Ovenproof frying pan or baking dish.

Instructions

1. Preheat the oven to 180°C regular bake.
2. Heat the oil and butter in a large frying pan. Season the chicken and brown well on both sides. Transfer to a plate. Add the bacon, leek, fennel, bay leaves, garlic and rosemary to the pan and cook for 5 minutes. Add the mushrooms, season and cook for another 5 minutes, turning frequently. Nestle the chicken into the vegetables along with any resting juices. Increase the heat and pour over the Marsala. Let it bubble up, then add the stock and bring back to the boil. Place in the oven and braise for 40 minutes, or until the chicken is cooked through.

30. Lamb Backstraps with Crushed Olives and Fennel Dressing

Prep Time: 15 Minutes

Cook Time: 45 Minutes

Serves: 6

Ingredients

- 4-6 boneless lamb backstraps, about 850 grams
- olive oil
- sea salt and ground pepper

Dressing:

- 1 teaspoon fennel seeds, toasted
- finely grated zest 1 lemon
- 2 tablespoons lemon juice
- 2 cloves garlic, crushed
- ¼ cup olive oil
- 2 tablespoons capers
- 1 tablespoon each finely chopped mint and parsley

To serve:

- 20 green olives, lightly crushed and pitted

Instructions

1. Brush the lamb with a little oil and season with salt and pepper.
2. Heat a large frying pan and when very hot, cook the lamb for about 2-3 minutes each side for medium-rare. Cooking time will depend on the thickness of the lamb. Try and get a good crust on the lamb. Transfer to a plate and rest, lightly covered, for
3. 5 minutes.
4. Dressing: Stir all the ingredients together in a bowl and season with salt and pepper.
5. To serve: Slice the lamb against the grain and place on a platter. Drizzle with the meat resting juices, then scatter over the olives and spoon over the dressing.